A Thread of HOPE

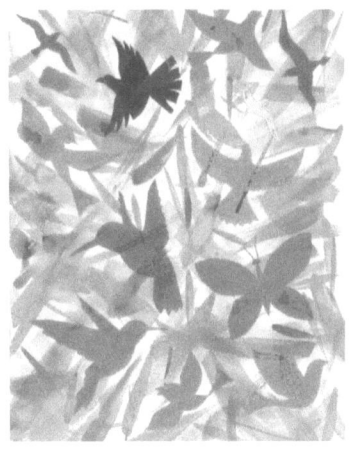

Denise Fletcher

Denise Fletcher

All rights reserved, no part of this publication may be reproduced by any means, electronic, mechanical photocopying, documentary, film or in any other format without prior written permission of the publisher.

Published by
Chipmunkapublishing
PO Box 6872
Brentwood
Essex CM13 1ZT
United Kingdom

http://www.chipmunkapublishing.com

Copyright © Denise Fletcher 2008

Edited by Danielle Atkins

Cover Design Copyright © 2008 by James Corbesia

A Thread of HOPE

About the Author

Denise Fletcher holds a degree in recreational therapy from Minnesota State University, Mankato and a massage practitioner certificate from the Minneapolis School of Massage. She struggles with bipolar disorder. Denise finds healing in the arts and writing is her passion. Her work has been published through On Edge, Kaleidoscope, Many Voices, Home Health Aide Digest, Hopekeeper's Magazine, Open Minds Quarterly, Bloomington Art Center and other various venues. She is currently a member of the Mental Health Consumer Survivor Network of Minnesota.

Denise Fletcher

A Thread of HOPE

Acknowledgements

Thanks to all the writers in my life for their inspiration and for being living examples. Namely, Sherri Connell, Lisa Copen, Gayle Darhower, Joanne Decker and C. Hope Clark. Also a special thanks to Dinah Laprairie for starting me on a career path as a writer.

Denise Fletcher

A Thread of HOPE

Description of the book:

Thread of Hope is more than a word salad. It reads like a zine exploring the boundaries of the mental illness system. This chapbook of semi-autobiographical poetry, prose and artistry demonstrates the healing power of creativity and spirituality in the life of the psychiatrized.

Denise Fletcher

A Thread of HOPE

Contents

- A Thread of Hope
- Butterfly Mountain
- Childhood Impressions
- Come Out Singing
- Craft Time
- Dear Doctor
- Exploring the World of Art
- Floating
- Free Bird
- Gambling Curse
- Haiku
- Haikus for Annie
- He Calls Me
- Hook, Line and Sinker
- I Can't Hear You God
- Impulses
- Letting Go
- Life's Highway
- Maybe I Want to Be Fat!
- Moods and Madness
- No Escape
- Northern Lights
- Peace
- Psychiatric Survivor
- Some Like it Hot
- Songbird
- The Art of Play
- The Days Be Done
- The Visit

Denise Fletcher

- The World is Ailing
- Time is Precious
- Wayfarer
- What are Friends For?
- About the Author
- Addendum

A Thread of HOPE

A Thread of Hope

Orphans on the streets
Crying out for love
Scrounging for a meal
And a warm place to sleep
Feeling lost and so afraid

Scanning for a friendly face
Hoping for someone to care
Wondering if their pain will end
Haunted by the memories
Of things they'd rather forget

Wishing for a miracle
Living on a Thread of Hope

The children are hungry
The children are crying
The children are beaten down,
Empty and cold,
The children are searching
For a safe refuge
And for a family
To have and to hold

Desperately wandering
Bruised and broken
Forced to turn a trick
Just to stay alive
Curious what tomorrow will bring

Treated like an animal

Denise Fletcher

Stranded, lost, forgotten
Living on the streets of fear
Waiting for anyone to reach out
To lend them a helping hand

Hoping for a miracle
Living on a Thread of Hope

The children are hungry
The children are crying
The children are beaten down,
Empty and cold,
The children are searching
For a safe refuge
And for a family
To have and to hold

Trying to remember a time
When life offered promise
Struggling for something more
Dreaming of a new day
In the land of hope

Praying for a miracle
Living on a Thread of Hope

A Thread of HOPE

Butterfly Mountain

Take me to a land
Where the children play
In sheer delight, running
With shrieks of laughter
Following the path of the butterfly
As they instinctively travel
Guided by sunlight
On their yearly journey
Through the seasons,
From egg to larva,
From pupa to butterfly
A kaleidoscope of colors
Clustered together in droves
On their endless search
For nectar and a bed of pines

Come fall the butterflies begin
Their three-day pilgrimage
Moving south with delicate wings
On their way to Butterfly Mountain
In Mexico's central valley
Pollinating plants along the way
Facing rain, cold and drought
Fearing loss of habitat
Flashing eyespots
Attracting a sparkling mate
Returning northward each spring
Celebrating their annual migration
With a new generation
Completing their 3000-mile trek

Denise Fletcher

Coming from far and wide
From the *Meadow* to the *Coast*
From the *Gulf* to the *Desert*
From the states to the forests
Arriving in good company
Like waves on Butterfly Mountain
Joined together by the millions
In a noble display
Of *Blues* and Purples
Of *Browns* and *Whites*
Of *Coppers* and *Sulphurs*
Both *Spotted* and *Painted*
As the insects take wing
On their voyage to freedom

The *Postman* delivers news of
The *Giant* gathering
The *Convict* with her *Hairstreak*
Beside both *Common* and *Great*
The *Skipper* with his *West Coast Lady*
Along with companions *Edith* and *Anna*
The *Viceroy* and *California Sister Julia*
The *Emperor* with *Lady Vanessa*
Joins the *Admiral* wearing his uniform
While escorting the *American Lady*
On their ascent to Butterfly Mountain
Where *Queen Victoria* resides
And the *Monarch* is king
And master of the *Milkweed*

A Thread of HOPE

*Note: Names that are in italic indicate the various types of butterflies.

Denise Fletcher

Childhood Impressions

Daily Reminder

Reminders of history are scattered around
Progress continues to abound

Inside

Mom making waffles before Sunday Mass
Scraps of fabric in the box, buttons in the tin
Hiding out in a makeshift tent of blankets
Digging through the presents in the closet

Vases full of lilacs around the kitchen
Pushing the cart at the grocery store
Baking, baking and more baking
Getting my teeth drilled, waiting for a sucker

Dad cooking up a fish fry in the black skillet
Doors slamming and radios blaring
Phone ringing off the hook
Magic mirrors in the funhouse
Rug burns from the wooden slide
Winning skeeball at the penny arcade

Loads of clothes to be folded on the couch
Blessing the ironing
Unopened mail on the coffee table
Newspapers bundled for the paper drive
Ashes in the fireplace
Buffing the wood floors until they shone

A Thread of HOPE

Outside

Icicles hanging from the gutters above the patio
Wood stacks on the side of the house
Plowing through a foot of snow
Seven children strewn about

Balls bouncing against the house walls
Rhubarb patches in the yard
Skipping school to catch sunrays, Station
Wagon in the driveway, salesman at the door

Biking to town for the latest read
Picnics at the Arboretum, hungry little ants
Walking barefoot on the rocky path to the shore
Swimming out to the buoy, jumping off the high dive
Screams coming from the roller coaster
Ferris wheel lights in the twilight

Church bazaars, cakewalks, parades and t-ball
Concert bands performing at the band shell
Climbing up the ladder to the tree house
Piles of leaves waiting to be bagged, Weeds
In the garden, snakes in the grass, Big Dipper
In the moonlight, North Star shining bright

Daily Reminder

Reminders of history are scattered around
Progress continues to abound

Denise Fletcher

Come Out Singing

I'm sitting at my kitchen table now looking out my window at the bright orange and red leaves on the trees in their fall array. It's hard for me to believe that over a year ago I was staring out the window of my hospital room looking at steel bars and concrete.

***

The steel doors separate me from the outside world. They are locked and there's no escape, except that door at the end of the corridor marked 'fire exit'. It crosses my mind that I can make a run for it, but I know that would be a complete waste of time. I'd been out that door before years ago and it hadn't been a fruitful experience. The loud sirens went off and I made a narrow escape out to the nearest highway, hitchhiking back home where I thought I would not only be safe, but free. No such luck; it was back to the psychiatric ward for me. How I hated being put under lock and key. Why in the world am I here?

My head is pounding; my mind is numb from all the anti-psychotic medications that are being pumped through my blood stream. My body is shaking from the side effects of all the toxic chemicals that are passing through my system. How I despise this wretched state. When a manic episode comes on, there's no stopping it. The brain is out of control. It's like being hit by a runaway train.

A Thread of HOPE

"Denise, your doctor's on his way," the nurse says to me.

"Follow me," my doctor says as we walk down the hall together to the meeting room. I take a seat across from him.

"Hey Doc, what's the results of my blood test today?" I ask.

Dr. A., in his usual humorous voice, replies, "You're leveling out just fine."

"Don't you ever go home?"

My psychiatrist seems to live at the hospital. He is either making his rounds on the ward or seeing other patients in his office. He works into the late hours of the night. When I do finally get to see him, it is usually not until nine in the evening.

"Too much work to do," he laughs, as I rub his shiny, bald head. Dr. A. always reminds me of Santa Claus with his fluffy beard and short stature.

"When am I going to get out of here?" I wonder aloud.

"In three to seven days," he says, as he makes his way out the door of the conference room and down the hall just as fast as he came.

Denise Fletcher

Darn, I forgot to ask for a pass for the following Saturday. My best friend is planning on taking me out to the pool for a swim. I'll have to wait another whole day, I thought to myself. He must have missed the note on my chart.

I wonder when my company is going to get here. The minutes seem like hours in a place like this, especially since I don't know anyone. All I can really do is sit and stare at the TV screen in the activity room. Once in a while I get lucky enough to find one other person that I can relate to and play a quick game of gin rummy.

"Denise, you have a guest," I hear the nurse call over the loudspeaker from her nursing station.

I rush down the hall from the activity room and there he is, as sure as the sun with his bright, cheerful smile.

"Hi Jim, am I ever glad to see you," I say as he gives me a big bear hug.

"I brought you a treat," he says and hands me a card and some candy along with my Bible. This time he even brought me a pair of pink slippers.

"What a surprise. Thanks so much," I reply.

"You'll be out of here in no time, don't worry," Jim says, as if he has read my mind.

A Thread of HOPE

I couldn't wait. "I just had some more blood tests," I show him as I rip the bandage and cotton ball off of my left arm. "I hate needles."

"I just saw your doctor on his way out and he wants us to see him together at his office next week," Jim tells me.

"That means I will be out of here soon, after all," I answer.

***

The cheers from the students watching the football team playing at the school down the street brings me back to reality. The sounds a few streets away are a sure sign of real life again. What a happy sound, I think to myself. It sure is nice being back home. At least now when I look out my window I know I am able to open it anytime to hear the melody of the songbirds calling in the oak trees. I am free to take a stroll around the park and watch the deer feeding. It makes all the difference in the world.

The memories of the hospital psychiatric wards still haunt me. I still have nightmares on occasion, but I've grown accustomed to taking my medication now for my medical condition. It sure beats going in and out of the hospital and living with frantic, racing thoughts and severe mood swings. It took a little over a year to get my life back on track and for my mind and my emotions to become stable again and it was well worth the effort. My psychiatrist can't believe my progress.

Back in his office I sit waiting for my appointment with Jim alongside me. The art in the room inspires me. It beats staring at the clock. I browse through a few magazines until Dr. A. calls my name. He doesn't even have to this time. I'm ready for him. He opens the door and gives the nod for me to come on in. Jim joins me. Jim takes a seat in the doctor's office, while I walk down the hall to hop on the scale. I don't even want to look at my weight. The medication is making me gain weight again. "I'm up a few pounds," I said, "I plan to walk every day, but I don't always get my exercise. Things come up."

Dr. A. knows all the secrets of living a long life. He's an expert on aging.

"Some women in Japan live until 124 years of age," he says.

"What's their secret?" I ask.

"Fish and kelp," he answers.

"I guess I better improve my diet then."

Back in the doctor's office, Dr. A. asks Jim, "How is she recovering so well?"

A Thread of HOPE

"Swimming," Jim answers.

Lots of prayer, I think to myself. The brain is a very fragile organ and I handle it with prayer. In my deepest, darkest hours I pray the Psalms and they comfort me. Why not, it worked for King David. He knew what it was like to live with a troubled spirit, and King David always *came out singing*.

Denise Fletcher

Craft Time

Certain people have a knack
Of creating homemade crafts.
My grandma, my sister and my best friend
Are gifted more than I can comprehend.

Come winter, spring, summer and fall
These people hear a special call.
To produce art for every occasion
No matter what the celebration.

A brain teeming with imagination
Doesn't wait for an invitation.
Art can be formed from any theme,
Creative minds conceive a dream.

All they need do is look around,
Materials can forever be found.
Wood, sand, rock, string and paper galore;
Bottles, beads, seashells, dried flowers and more.

An inch of ribbon, a sprinkle of lace
Add that special touch of grace.
A bureau full of crayons, a drawer filled with paints,
Children waiting to be inspired by the saints.

My home is filled with simple gifts

A Thread of HOPE

Not for sale and given with a kiss.
Just come on in and glance around,
See what one-of-a-kind creations abound.

Ornaments of toothpick stars decorate the tree,
A shingled manger scene to worship the Trinity.
Freshly applied shellac and the sweet smell of pine,
A musical box, wood clocks and feeders divine.

A beach in a bottle, splat art greeting cards,
Hanging seashell mobiles enough to fill a yard.
Rose-painted eggs blown out Ukrainian style
Searching high and low and stretching to a mile.

A wind vane riding in the summer breeze
Doesn't take kindly to the bugs or the bees.
A translucent windsock torn to shreds by the storm
Tells us it's time to go inside and keep warm.

A miniature planetarium in the dark;
Stars on the ceiling reflecting a spark.
A silhouetted lighthouse in the night
Painted black with a spot of white.

A man of playing cards walking a tightrope
Searching for a thread of hope.
A face relief of plasters Paris,
Giving his life a touch of merit.

Denise Fletcher

Specially carved and painted pumpkins
With candy served to little bumpkins
Circuit boards draped to his overalls;
The most outrageous costume of all.

Painted rocks on the windowsill,
Reminding us to learn to be still.
Bookmarks laminated to order
Fits the bill in the book border.

Models of speckled-painted butterflies;
Always watching for those bargain buys.
Given the right tools of the trade,
Just imagine what can be made.

Strong loving hands fashioned these designs,
A future full of promise, one of many great minds.
Unprecedented inventions of every shape and size;
Something new and different deserving of a prize.

A Thread of HOPE

Dear Doctor!

You are quick to call this mental illness
A chemical imbalance or a brain disease,
But have you ever thought to check me for
An allergy or a vitamin deficiency?

You are anxious to point out my anxiety
And label me with PTSD, OCD or BAD,
When what I really need is to eat my vegetables
And exercise to increase my BAT*.

You are happy to prescribe me an antidepressant,
So I take my chill pill every day as you requested.
Just remember this next time you write out that slip:
I am a child of God not a subject to be tested.

My parents tell me to "listen to the doctor",
But which one might that be?
The one who profits off drugs or the
Doctor who teaches vitamin therapy?

"Take your medication" they all chime in
My parents, my siblings, my friends,
But what they all neglect to realize is the
The drugs are a means to an "end".

My parents tell me to "listen to the doctor",
But which one might that be?
The one who sentences me to ill health,
Or the doc who inspires me to be free?

You know labels do more harm than good,

Denise Fletcher

Yet you stick me with this "brain disease"
And now that I am tagged I will have to
Spend the rest of my life being teased.

I am not alone you say, there are many others
"Like me", the list goes on and on you see.
There's Vivien Leigh, Patty Duke, Kay Jamison,
And more, the latest being Jane Pauley.

Sadly, many people are woefully misdiagnosed,
Such as Frances Deitrick who had a brain tumor.
Physical problems masquerade as mental problems,
And others are tragically diagnosed according to rumor.

I see the likes of me portrayed on television,
In the media, and on the silver screen, yet
Hollywood can't get past those old reflections
Of the "Golden Era" that are just plain mean.

I'm no genius and I'm no freak, but
I may have some creative tendencies.
Those gifts originate from God alone,
Not generated by some brain disease.

(*BAT = Brown Adipose Tissue)

A Thread of HOPE

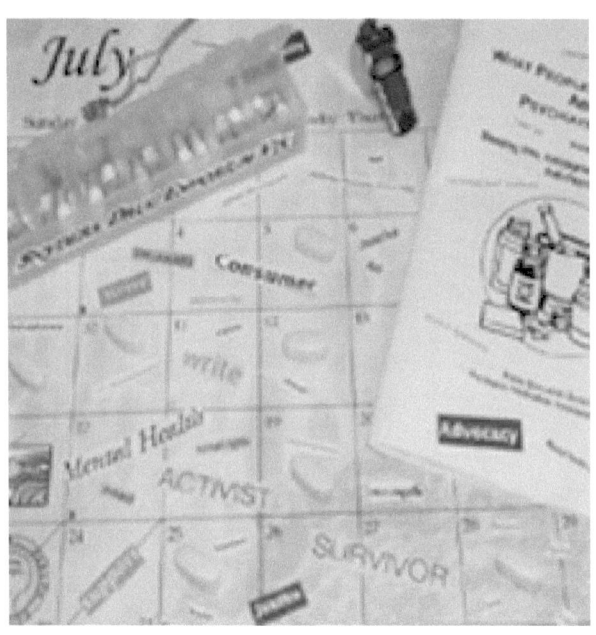

Denise Fletcher

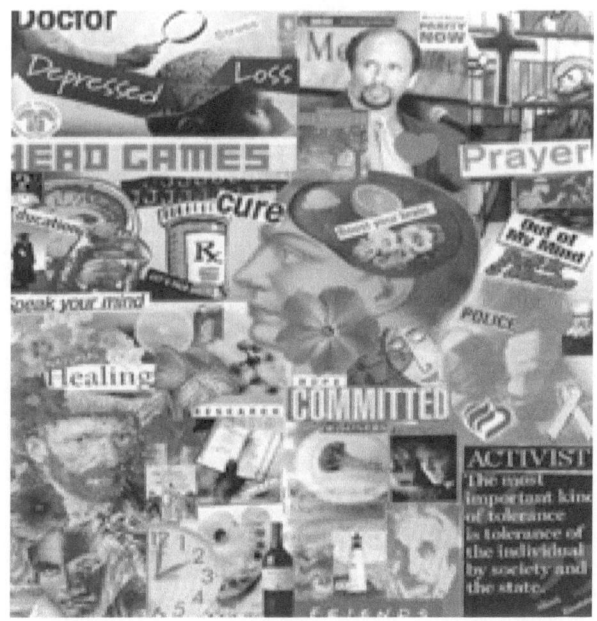

Committed

A Thread of HOPE

Exploring the World of Art

In a world gone awry, art can become a welcome release from your troubles and is a very important part of healing from trauma. Art is both fun and relaxing and a great stress reliever. Art can be utilized as a method not only to express your deepest thoughts and feelings, but as a tool to get to know yourself better and to discover your hidden talents. Create art for art's sake. Art does not always have to be for public consumption, competition or for material gain. Art should definitely not be used as a way for others to analyze your psyche. If your art is very personal, it may be best to use discretion and share it only with trusted friends or family. Ask others you know for their personal perspectives on art, but do not let them discourage you from exploring new modes of personal expression. Make it your goal to try your hand at something new and different that you've never done before.

When determining what types of art that you would like to pursue, you may consider exploring the world of art by visiting your local community center or art gallery. Take a good look around your community to get a sense of where your interests may lie. Art takes many forms, such as sculptures in the park, flower gardens, rock formations, and paintings, drawings or photos hanging on the walls of Churches, libraries or local restaurants. Other valuable resources for various ideas are craft and fabric stores, bookstores, or art supply stores.

Denise Fletcher

Taking a walk in the woods or walking along the beach will stir your imagination and may bring out the collector in you. Shells, rocks, petrified wood and other assorted nature items are great resources for craft projects like mobiles or collages. The more you observe your environment, the more you will become attuned to the many art forms available to you. Even baking cakes or cookies can become an art form!

It is always helpful to take a class to learn a new skill and art is no exception. There are many opportunities for classes through art centers, community colleges, or even at craft stores, depending on the level of your interest and skill. If finances are a problem, then consider checking out art books or videotapes at the nearest library. There are innumerable experts who have written how-to books on many different art forms, such as jewelry, woodworking, quilting, computer graphics, etc. You can learn almost anything you want to know in self-help books. If you live in a large city, there are large Institutes of Art, which are open to the public where you can tour exhibits by world-renowned artists. These displays change with the seasons and are full of amazing works of art that bring fresh ideas no matter how many times you visit.

Find a relaxed atmosphere such as a coffee shop or reading room and bring a spiral notebook or journal with you to jot down notes. Challenge yourself to write a short poem or song on

A Thread of HOPE

something that is of value to you. Give yourself some personal time to reflect on your creative goals. Contemplate such questions as:

What types of art do I like most? Least?
What methods of art would I like to learn?
What is my primary interest? Secondary?
What subjects would I like to concentrate on most? Least?
What points do I want to convey?
What is the best way to express a particular point?
What motivates me to create art the most? Least?
What are my future goals?

Write your own questions related to art and write down your answers in your notebook. Your questions and answers will change over time. Keeping an art journal is a good way to measure your progress. If you are proficient in a particular skill, which you would like to share, you may consider teaching a class or volunteering with a non-profit agency, which specializes in the healing arts. My challenge to you is to embrace your inner child by doing any creative activity, which brings you joy and which helps you to focus on the present moment.

Denise Fletcher

Floating

Floating off to sleep
    Half asleep half awake
Living in my dream world
Where my mind escapes
    At peace
    At rest
Releasing all my cares
    To the clouds

Floating off to sleep
    Half asleep half awake
Living in my dream world
I feel myself falling
    My body shakes
I startle myself
    My mind wakes

Floating off to sleep
    Half awake half asleep
Living in my dream world
Forgetting the day's troubles
    Freeing my mind
    From the pain
Letting go

Floating off to sleep
    Half awake half asleep
Living in my dream world
    Blissful rest
    Blissful peace

A Thread of HOPE

Free Bird

I'm a free bird
Floating through the sky
I'm a free bird
Watching birds go by
I'm a free bird
Feeling with my wings
I'm a free bird
Watching everything

> One day I'll see
> The great things I was meant to see
> One day I'll be
> A vessel for His Majesty

I'm a free bird
Flying through the sky
I'm a free bird
Knowing I can fly
I'm a free bird
Swaying in the breeze
I'm a free bird
Come to rest upon the tree

> One day I'll see
> The great things I was meant to see
> One day I'll be
> A vessel for His Majesty

I'm a free bird
Going high as I can be

Denise Fletcher

I'm a free bird
Viewing all that I can see
I'm a free bird
Hoping that one day
I'll be a free bird
Latching onto higher things

A Thread of HOPE

Gambling Curse

The full moon pulls me
To the glittering lights
Music fills the air
Smoke is everywhere
Coins clink into the tray
Beckoning me to play
It's a carnival of mystery
Will I win or will I lose?
Man versus machine
The same old struggle
This time I lose
Next time I choose

Denise Fletcher

Haiku

Off to the movies
Hope it is a blockbuster
Surely not a dud

A Thread of HOPE

Haikus for Annie*

Mother Lioness
A Champion of Children
Annie the Stallion

Hurricane Annie
Speaking from California
One Power Talker

*Dedicated to Dr. Annie Armen

Denise Fletcher

He Calls Me

He calls me to the rocks
to come and seek His face
I can see Him in the wind,
the waves, the trees.
I can see Him in the birds,
I can see Him in the sky
and I can see Him in the
changing of the leaves.

He is so lovely,
He is so lovely,
He is so lovely each day I see.
He is so lovely,
He is so lovely,
He is so lovely to me.

A Thread of HOPE

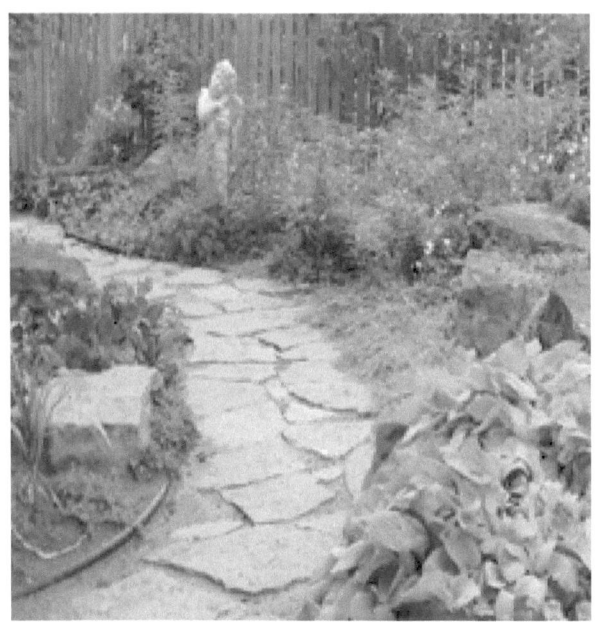

Healing Garden

Denise Fletcher

Hook, Line and Sinker

Whenever I even hear the word fishing, the first thing that comes to my mind is my dear old Dad. Ever since I was a little girl, all I ever remember my Dad wanting to do in his spare time was to go fishing. He was fishing long before I was ever born. Fishing is in his blood. He must have learned it from his Dad, because Grandpa was an expert too. His freezer was a tribute to that.

My Dad drove a hard bargain. If I wanted to be with him, which I did, then I would have to learn how to fish. A major part of learning how to fish meant catching our own live bait! My Dad used to take my brothers and sisters and I out to the marshes to chase after frogs. My Dad was always sending us out after the heavy rains to dig up the bait. We would get up at the crack of dawn and have to beat the robins to the night crawlers that were popping their heads up in the grass.

I always wanted to drag along, but being from a large family, only so many people could fit in the boat. On the rare occasions that I did get to ride along, I was always a clumsy oaf and squirmed at the sight of the squiggly worms and tiny minnows. I abhorred having to put their lives on the line. To this day, I still hate hooking those pesky little creatures.

There were times my Dad would want to take the whole family out for the day. One of his favorite

A Thread of HOPE

spots to fish was under the bridge at what was known as the Narrows. We'd be all lined up like a can of sardines along the shore. I wish some of Dad's gift would have rubbed off on me, but even now, every time I go fishing I feel like an accident waiting to happen.

For instance, there was the time I was fishing at a city lake. Instead of catching the muskie in the mouth with a hook, I ended up snagging the line around its neck. I panicked and handed my friend, Jim my fishing pole, which he continued to reel in. When Jim got the fish to shore, the noose slipped off and the fish was flipping on the waterline. We didn't have a net, so Jim used his hands to grab the gills and brought it in. Thank goodness Jim was there or we wouldn't have been eating that night!

I've heard about dogs taking their owners for walks, but I never knew this could apply to fish. One day, Jim and I decided to drag our gear out to a county park for the day. I thought it would be a typical day of fishing, so I decided to just let the fishing take care of itself. I hooked the worm and cast out the line and then laid my pole down on the dock waiting for bait. I rolled up my shirtsleeves and my pant legs and stretched back, hoping to grab a quick tan.

The next thing I knew, my fishing pole was in the water and I was swimming after it! The Sunny had yanked the pole clear off the dock! Darned if I was going to lose my pole to a fish. When I finally

Denise Fletcher

reached my pole, I felt a pull on the line. I told Jim and he yelled, "reel 'em in!" When I finally did reach the shore, my clothes were soaking wet, but the Sunny was still on the line! For the remainder of the day, Jim and I were catching Sunnies left and right. They were the biggest Sunnies I'd ever seen. We both caught our limit that day.

I'll never forget the time I almost gouged Jim's eye out! I doubt Jim will ever forget either. We were fishing along the north shore of Minnesota and went out to the flat rocks. Jim was far more experienced than I was and encouraged me to set up and cast out on my own. As soon as I reached backward to cast my pole out farther, the 3-hooked rappela stuck into Jim's cheek right below his left eye.

I wasn't paying attention and I hadn't noticed that he had been standing right behind me. Lucky for him he screamed loud enough to alert me to the disaster before I yanked my pole. It's a miracle that Jim didn't end up in the hospital ER that day. I can't blame Jim for being squeamish whenever I even mention the word "fishing".

A Thread of HOPE

I Can't Hear You God

I can't hear you God
Above the clutter of the world
Above the contradictions of doctrines
Above the noise and confusion
And arguments of family quarrels,
God where can I go to listen
God I thank you that I can hear you
Amidst the flowers and the trees
God I can hear your voice
In the whisper of the wind
And the changing of the autumn leaves
God I can see you in the golden
Sunshine on the rolling hills
And in the morning sunrise
You are saying, 'see how beautiful
This world really is'
God I thank you that your voice
Is coming out loud and clear

Denise Fletcher

Impulses

A sense of surprise
A matter of sex appeal
An impulsive desire
Done without any forethought
Planned with no intent
But hidden satisfaction
The wonder of fulfillment
And instant pleasure
Feeling his body next to mine
Soft and warm
A delight to achieve
Feeling beautiful again.

A Thread of HOPE

Letting Go

Your message came out loud and clear
my place was there with you
No right to have a life of my own
No option to choose
only to go where I was needed
when I was told
irregardless of my circumstances
No matter the personal cost
even if God called me somewhere else
you said NO
all because you couldn't let go

Restless and wandering
I needed to be free
I wanted to run like the wind
Fly like a bird
but I was given no choice
Feeling trapped like an animal
never allowed to roam
Too far on my own
unable to make my own mistakes
put under constant pressure
with prying eyes watching
watching my every move

Forgetting that I have
a mind of my own
A heart yearning for more
Eyes to see the world
Ears to hear the truth

Denise Fletcher

A mouth to speak up
No longer afraid of you
and the grasp you held on my life
A body no longer bound
by your plans for me
A spirit that is free
A soul that remains searching
searching for my place
In the scheme of things
a sacred space where I belong
in the kingdom of God
finally learning to let go

A Thread of HOPE

Life's Highway

Traveling down life's highway
The future unfolds
In your visions
And your dreams
Dreams fade
Reality strikes
Visions die
Responsibilities seep in
All you've strived for
Gone
Wasted
On precious time
Scarcely a moment left
To enjoy
All the fruits
Of your labor

Denise Fletcher

Maybe I Want To Be Fat!

Maybe I want to be fat!
Did you ever think of that?
Maybe I want to be fat
just to piss you off.
Maybe I want to stay
in my protective shell.
Maybe I like being stared at
and stared down
and called names
and brought down to the ground
and kicked around
just to make you
feel better about yourself
every time
you call me a name
or give me that look
like
gawd woman
Can't you take care of yourself?
How do you look at yourself
in the mirror every morning?
Don't you even care?

Excuse me for living --
Excuse me for enjoying
the simple pleasures of life,
like -- eating.
Excuse me for wanting to feel
normal -- for once.
Excuse me for wanting to live.
What do you want anyway?

A Thread of HOPE

Would you rather I starved myself
just to satisfy your need
of never having to look
at another fat person again?

Sorry if my excess poundage
is a little too much
for your eyes to bear.
Sorry if I have to eat to live
even if you think
that I live to eat --
no matter what you say.
You think that what
you see on the outside
is how I really feel on the inside?
You think I would want to be
Perfect
like YOU
if I could?
Don't be silly --
God help us all if we have to be
the same.

Who asked you anyway?
No one asked me
what shape I wanted to be
or what form
I would like to take.
Don't you think I would
choose
to be normal
to fit in
to be accepted?

Denise Fletcher

NO WAY --
Maybe --
just maybe,
I like who I am.
Life can't always be
the way we want.
We hope.
We change.
We fight to survive
and after all this,
I am still happy to be
ALIVE
as a W-O-M-A-N

A Thread of HOPE

Moods and Madness

My life is relegated
    By moods and madness
Emotional ups
        And
            Downs
Feel the feelings
    Face the fear
Wake up
    It's a new day

Feel the feelings
    Face the fear
Be glad to be alive
    Try something new

Be creative
    Explore
        Experiment
Imagine
    Conceive
        Achieve

Reach out to someone
    Make a friend
Share your feelings
    Express yourself

Face rejection
    Believe in yourself
Overcome self-doubt
    Know your worth

Denise Fletcher

Make yourself known
     Be a friend
Feel the feelings
     Face the fear

A Thread of HOPE

No Escape

His gentle young self peers up at him
half man, half skeleton
trying to bring him back to reality
he cannot escape those walls
his soul is lost to his dreams
he is trapped inside the loft
of broken dolls and no one seems
to be able to break through
save his young spirit as he roams
his apartment trying to reach him

Denise Fletcher

Northern Lights

If by some chance we meet,
under the heavenly night
my gaze will be as bright
as the northern lights.
My love for you as deep
as the great expanse of space.

If by some chance we meet,
in a distant day or place,
my heart will be as strong
as a newly forming star.
My love for you as long
as the great expanse of time.

A Thread of HOPE

Peace

Peace is silence
A resting silence
When all is still...and peaceful
Sitting with your loved one
On an empty beach at daybreak
Listening to the waves break on the shore
Gazing at the moon
Lying in bed at midnight
Half awake, glaring at the ceiling's
Funny shapes from the moonlight
Showing through the silky curtain
Feeling the cool breeze coming through
The partially opened window
Or even...
Resting in front of the fireplace
On the soft carpet with a pillow
Beneath your head
Listening to the cackle of the fire
Mixed with some Bach symphony orchestra
Music playing on the stereo

Denise Fletcher

Psychiatric Survivor

I've been locked up
Locked down

Drugged up
Pushed around

Shut up
Shut down

Chained up
Strapped down

Court-ordered
Dragged around

Scapegoated
Tracked down

Profiled
And blacklisted

Yet through it all
By the Grace of God

I survive

A Thread of HOPE

Some Like it Hot

Venturing out into new territory is exciting, but the winding road in the middle of Oregon country never seemed to end. My stomach was churning and my mind wandering. My best friend Jim and I had just moved to the Oregon coast and we wanted to explore more of the scenic beauty. Jim had driven five hours as we reached the town of Detroit, southeast of Salem. Once settled into our motel, we suited up and headed out to Breitenbush just a few miles away.

After parking the Chevy Luv, we strolled down the trail towards the gift shop to purchase our day passes. Unbeknownst to us when we arrived, the staff had failed to notify us that clothes are optional! Nothing had prepared us for this, but we weren't going to let that stop us from enjoying the natural hot springs or the magnificent view of the ancient forest. We roamed around the historic lodge, read in the sanctuary, and snapped some photos before basking in the sun. I slowly stepped into the hot springs. The water was so hot; it took all I could muster to put my whole body in. Sinking into the water felt like a dream and healing to the bones. Once nestled back into the crevice of the rocks, Jim and I were able to make conversation with our fellow sojourners.

Jim spotted it first. The all-natural wood structure was striking. Growing up with a sauna, I certainly couldn't pass it up. We both exited the pools and sauntered over to the small hut where another visitor was bathing. After a healthy sweat in the sauna, I cooled off in the showers while Jim hopped into the tub. I felt a little uncomfortable at first walking around all those naked bodies, but after a few hours of rest and relaxation, I became more at ease in the environment.

After four hours of bathing and hiking around the trails, we were hungry. We were anxious to taste their vegetarian cuisine. As we made our way to the lunchroom, we joined the guests in line and took our split pea soup and drink to the lodge table. We enjoyed the sounds of children's laughter and friendly conversations over simmering peppermint tea. The peppermint definitely helped to settle my stomach and calm my nerves. Some of the other visitors asked us where we were from and we reciprocated. There was nothing like hot steaming herbal tea to bring out the inner stirrings of the heart. After a long morning, it was time to leave. It had been great to be in such a peaceful setting with soothing streams of running water around the entire retreat center. As Jim was driving South towards Detroit, I knew that Breitenbush would forever be etched in my memory.

A Thread of HOPE

Songbird

Up before the crack of dawn
The nestling sings its melody
At home high in the branches
She announces a new day

Denise Fletcher

The Art of Play

Learning the art of play means developing a playful attitude while working with your client. This not only helps the client, but it is essential in dealing with the mundane daily tasks that, at times become very frustrating. The daily chores of planning menus, preparing meals, cleaning, and personal care can be both exhausting and time-consuming.

Although the main objective of the hospice or home health aide is to help and assist the client as much as possible and to ease their pain, these duties should not deter you from the chance you have to learn and grow together in a partnership. Ask your client to make a list of their hobbies and interests, along with future goals that they would like to pursue. Encourage them to dream. Get to know your client as a person, their likes and dislikes and develop ways that you can engage them in creative and meaningful activities. This will help divert their focus away from their chronic illness and/or chronic pain.

The more your client can participate alongside you, the better they will feel. This will also make your work more fulfilling. Some of my most rewarding times with my clients were spent replanting flowers or baking bread together. Seek out fun ways to bring comfort to your client's lives through arts, crafts, literature, music or anything that is soothing. To bring spice into the life of your client, you can

A Thread of HOPE

play a variety of music from bluegrass to reggae, cook something different for a cultural experience, post inspirational quotes on the refrigerator and keep both the environment clean and the surroundings cheerful.

While stretching your client's limbs, help them to stretch their minds as well with stimulating conversation by sharing jokes or discussing current events. If you are a hospice aide and your client is bedridden from a terminal illness, you can obtain music or audio CDs from the library, read poetry, encourage them to write their memoirs or create a scrapbook. This will help them invoke happy memories in their lives.

Assist your client at whatever stage of their disabling medical condition and teach them to pace themselves. It is important that they know their limits. Caregivers need to understand and acknowledge the physical and/or emotional pain of the person they are assisting. It is especially common for anyone living with a chronic illness to deal with depression.

When I have experienced depression, it feels like I am driving in a fog and am unable to see the road ahead. It is difficult to concentrate. At times I feel like I am heading for a crash and I need to pull over to take time out until I can see the road ahead once again. If you notice that your client is persistently sad, has decreased energy, increased irritability or irregular changes in diet or sleep habits, do your best to draw them out with compassion and gentleness. Do not force intervention, but help your client remain focused on the moment by engaging in healthy, positive conversation. Maintaining your equilibrium and keeping a positive and cheerful attitude is essential.

If their depression persists, ask them to speak with their nurse or doctor about their feelings and their treatment options. Treatment for depression and/or manic-depression can range from herbal supplements to prescription medication to light, massage, and talk or vitamin therapy. There is a wide range of options, depending on whether their practitioner is traditional or naturopathic.

Not only is it good for the aide to know the symptoms of depression and available treatment options, it is important to be aware of the possible harmful side effects of prescription medication. If the client is experiencing severe adverse side effects, such as shaking or dyskinesia, exhort them to share this information with their nurse or doctor immediately. It is extremely important that your client is receiving a proper dosage of medication. Encourage them to become their own advocate and to speak up and speak out. Although it is not your job to disseminate medication, it is your responsibility to assist your client in maintaining a nourishing quality of life while they are in your personal care.

A Thread of HOPE

Finding ways to keep life upbeat is the key to being a valuable hospice or home health aide. Advise your client to relieve stress and anxiety by listening to relaxing and calming music, talking to supportive friends, reading a daily devotional, eating a healthy diet, writing in a journal, walking in a garden or any of a number of coping skills that will guide them through the rocky path of life.

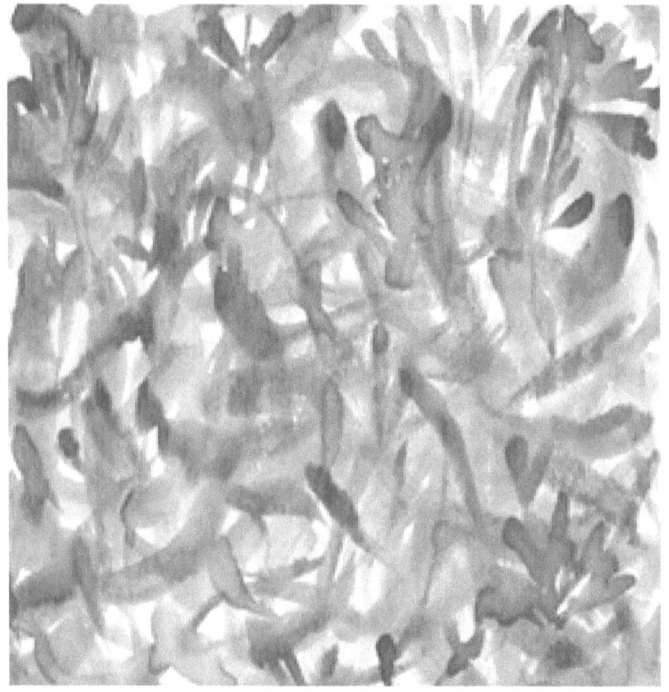

Springtime

Denise Fletcher

The Days Be Done

Our days are over
Rest is won
Let us go now
Sleep will come
Tiring, exhausting,
Restless days
Let us go now
Sleep will come
The days be done
We had our fill
May we rest now
Sleep will come

A Thread of HOPE

The Need for Choice

It is my experience that the mental health system is being used to discredit people and takes away our basic human rights. Ever since the eugenics movement, persons with mental illness have been considered "mental defectives". The stigma of the mental illness label does not go away. According to the Merriam Webster Dictionary, "Stigma" is defined as "a mark to discredit or shame".

The stigma of the mental illness label is so prevalent in our society today that anyone who is branded "mentally ill" is deemed "crazy" and considered potentially "dangerous". The corporate media perpetuates this myth with their sensationalistic reporting that anyone labeled "mentally ill" is to be feared.

It is fear that drives the mental health system. It is fear that causes forced drugging and forced involuntary electroshock. It is fear that keeps people with mental illness locked up. It is fear that even now is causing drug implants of powerful and toxic time-released anti-psychotic medications to be manufactured to be used on anyone labeled mentally ill that does not comply with this forced drug regime.

No longer does the mental health professional need our permission to drug us. This ought not to be so. Is there no room for compromise in the mental health system? The mental health practitioners

Denise Fletcher

think that if we don't agree with their drug regimen, that they have the right to take away our basic human rights. Our right to make an educated, informed decision about our own treatment for our own medical condition, whatever the case may be. I understand that force is sometimes necessary in certain precarious situations, but only for a limited time and only for safety reasons.

Although very few insurance companies cover alternative treatments at this time, individual consumers need to know we have a right to choose whatever treatment we deem appropriate, as anyone else would with any other medical condition. Using safe alternative treatments for mental health conditions should be a personal decision between you and your physician or practitioner, not made by a family member or a spouse. Family members need to support consumer/survivors in their choices and respect their decisions.

I am a strong believer in Holistic Health and Integrative Medicine. I need to know I have choices in my treatment. I choose life and the anti-psychotic medications do not enhance my quality of life. In the past I have been forced to be on heavy anti-psychotic and neuroleptic drugs and they can and do cause neurological damage.

After taking the anti-psychotic medications for a few brief months over the course of merely three years, I have already begun to exhibit early signs of

A Thread of HOPE

Parkinson's disease and tardive dyskinesia. Prolixin depletes dopamine in the brain, which in turn causes dyskinesia and the shakes. This medication has caused me to have tremors for weeks, shaking at all hours of the day and night making it very difficult for me to sit still and nearly impossible to sleep. I experienced severe restlessness and pacing. My head pounds and my mind goes numb. The medication has caused my hair to fall out, severe weight gain, and memory loss and has also caused deterioration of brain cells. Zyprexa has been reported to cause diabetes. Klonopin decreases white blood cells in the blood stream, which weakens the immune system. Worst of all, the anti-psychotic medication makes me feel spiritually dead inside, which is devastating to one's spirit.

I will not deny the fact that prescription drugs are necessary when the brain is not functioning properly. The medication helps to slow my mind down from a manic episode and I do believe it is important to take medication for mental illness, but I think the prescription drugs should be used sparingly and with extreme caution. There should be a definite limit on the amount of drugs prescribed per day, in my opinion.

People diagnosed with a mental illness should have a right to know the long-term side effects of the prescription drugs that we are taking. By taking away our right to choose our own treatment, we are being denied our basic human right to make an

Denise Fletcher

educated, informed decision about our own treatment for *our own medical condition.* There are many safe and healthy alternative vitamins and supplements available on the market today that will enhance mental health and enable consumers to live longer and feel healthier. * All consumer/survivors should have the right to choose safe and healthy alternatives, such as vitamin therapy, if they so choose, *without fear of reprisal.*

Patch Adams said it best when he said, "We need to start treating the patient as well as the disease."

Note: Since writing this article, I have found a psych doctor who has helped me come off the neuroleptics, kept my doses low, and prescribed multi-vitamins. Now all the shaking is gone! I am on the road to recovery!

A Thread of HOPE

The Visit

I stopped by today
You didn't recognize me
The drugs have taken their toll
On your body, mind and soul

It hurts me to see you
Pacing up and down the hall
Struggling to find a place to sit
With those restless legs

It hurts me to see you
With scars on your wrists
I reached out to touch you
But you pushed me away

It hurts me to see you
Shaking in the chair
Staring at the TV screen
Not saying a word

It hurts me to see you
Being spoon fed by the nurse
Drooling as you eat
Your soup and crackers

It hurts me to see you
Sleeping with ratted hair
On yellow-stained sheets
Unshaven and undone

I stopped by today

Denise Fletcher

You didn't recognize me
The drugs have taken their toll
On your body, mind and soul

A Thread of HOPE

The World Is Ailing

The World is ailing fast today
It breeds contempt and war.
The fighting never ceases,
But the pains truly endure.

Senseless murder on the streets,
Raises crying from the womb.
All too common is the bloodshed
Of their precious loves ones.

There is no quick panacea
That can heal the broken lives
And broken hearts
Of helpless humans.

Denise Fletcher

Time is Precious

My heart is breaking.
My heart is torn.
My heart is damaged beyond repair.
Time can not always mend my broken heart.
Time is Precious.

My soul is searching.
My soul is restoring.
My soul is healing the damage done.
Time will tell if my soul will mend.
Time is precious.

My mind is anxious.
My mind is distressed.
My mind is afflicted and needs repair.
Time will renew my mind's woes.
Time is precious

A Thread of HOPE

Wayfarer

I'm just a traveler
Passing through
Always waiting for something
More exciting to do
Always looking for some
Needy soul to cheer
And hoping that my joy
Will shine through

Denise Fletcher

What are Friends For?

If I can't call you up
When I'm down
What are friends for?

If I can't cheer you up
When you frown
What are friends for?

If I can't make you laugh
When you cry
What are friends for?

If I can't say hello
When you say goodbye
What are friends for?

A Thread of HOPE

Recovery

```
E  I  Y  S  N  I  M  A  T  I  V  M  O  C  E
P  E  D  T  J  D  D  R  D  N  Y  A  P  I  R
M  U  I  E  I  O  X  S  A  V  N  F  H  S  U
X  A  F  V  C  K  K  C  Y  C  O  T  K  U  T
E  N  E  T  O  I  A  R  E  S  A  C  P  M  A
D  T  O  E  B  M  T  H  Y  L  I  M  A  F  N
N  R  F  D  A  E  F  E  C  Y  C  H  E  C  D
E  R  O  A  O  G  X  E  T  A  N  H  Y  T  Y
I  H  O  P  V  K  K  I  W  T  S  D  O  O  F
R  L  A  M  R  F  N  A  C  P  I  V  I  E  W
F  T  V  C  U  U  L  C  R  I  B  W  O  V  D
O  D  I  N  M  H  W  E  N  T  O  E  O  E  T
A  S  L  M  P  E  T  S  A  J  O  A  E  R  C
E  H  O  U  S  I  N  G  F  O  K  L  M  Y  F
E  C  E  R  A  Y  K  R  O  S  S  F  O  M  D
```

ACTIVISM	ADVOCACY	ART
ATTITUDE	BOOKS	CHARITY
COMMUNITY	DANCE	DOCTOR
EXERCISE	FAMILY	FOODS
FRIENDS	HOBBIES	HOUSING
HUMOR	MASSAGE	MOVIES
MUSIC	NATURE	PETS
POETRY	PRAYER	SLEEP
THERAPY	TRAVEL	VITAMINS

Denise Fletcher

Addendum

Previously Published

A Thread of Hope, Poetry Sharings Journal, August 2004
Childhood Impressions, NISA Writers Circle Online, March 2005
Come Out Singing, NISA Writers Circle Online, May 2004
Committed, On Edge, Issue #3, Fall 2006
Dear Doctor, Doctor Yourself e-news, Vol. 6, No. 4, March 2006
Exploring the World of Art, Many Voices, Vol. XVIII, No. 5, October 2006
Floating, Poetry Sharings Journal, January 2001
Haiku, Poetry Sharings Journal, October 2004
Healing Garden, On Edge, Issue #4, Spring 2007
Hook Line and Sinker, Open Minds Quarterly, Winter 2005
Impulses, On the Threshold of a Dream, Vol. III, 1992
Letting Go, On Edge, Issue #4, Spring 2007
Life's Highway, Echoes of Yesterday, Winter 1994
Moods and Madness, NISA Writers Circle Online, September 2005
No Escape, Charaka Revue, Vol. 4, Issue 2, May 2003
Northern Lights, NISA Writers Circle Online, August 2004

A Thread of HOPE

Peace, Zephrus IV, 1974
Psychiatric Survivor, Open Minds Quarterly, Summer 2006
Recovery collage, Open Minds Quarterly, Summer 2007
Songbird, Kaleidoscope, Issue #54, Winter/Spring 2007
The Art of Play, Home Health Aide Digest, July/August 2005
The Days Be Done, Bloomington Art Center, Seasons, September 2006
The Need for Choice, Cry Justice Conference, 2003
The Visit, CSN Recovery Connection, Winter 2006/2007
The World is Ailing, Seasons to Come, Spring 1995
What are Friends For? NISA Writers Circle Online, November 2005

Denise Fletcher

www.ingramcontent.com/pod-product-compliance
Ingram Content Group UK Ltd.
Pitfield, Milton Keynes, MK11 3LW, UK
UKHW041413180426
11947UKWH00007B/98